HEALTHY EATING HABITS

BEST WHAT TO EAT NUTRITION HACKS

Dr. PASINDU ABEYSUNDARA

(MBBS-SRI LANKA)

The information provided in this book is designed to complement but not replace, the relationship between a patient and his/her physician. Any person above age 18 can use this information unless it has a very serious health concern.

Moreover, the information provided here should not be used over the professional opinion of the own physician of a patient with a particular illness that needs a continual and follow-up treatment for that illness although the information provided here may aid in the management of that illness directly or indirectly.

Table of Contents

Foreword

There is a common saying that "You are what you eat".

It is far more relevant to these times as the prevalence of cancer and other non-communicable diseases like diabetes, heart disease, stroke, etc. are rising day by day. Research says that these illnesses have a strong association with your diet.

Thus, consuming a diet with healthy groups of food in adequate amounts will permit a healthy life. But what should we eat?

There are lots of benefits of eating healthy that include, Weight loss, lowering cholesterol, blood pressure, having a functional and good-looking body, boosting your immunity, having protection from non-communicable diseases and cancer, promoting a healthy and happy mind, etc.

You can't achieve any of these unless you are taking a nutritious and proper diet, rich in all the nutrients that your body needs.

This book explains the best healthy eating tips and plans with their health benefits driving you one step towards healthy eating motivation for a happy and disease-free life.

Similarly, the author explains these, based on scientifically proven facts in a simple and easy-to-understand manner.

Thus, this book makes one of the best nutrition and diet-related books in the market guiding you to answer the question "What to eat to be healthy?"

Chapter 1.

What is a Balanced Diet: The Greatest Dietary Hack You Need to Know!

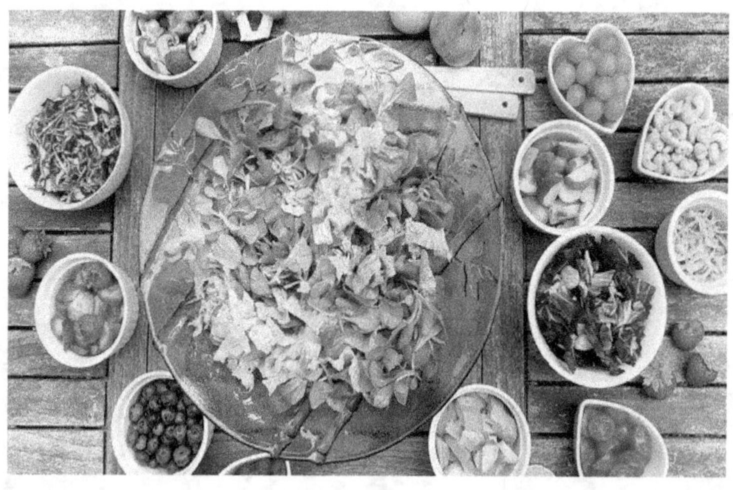

Nutrition is one of the most important subjects to people of all ages. That is because malnutrition will result in many devastating consequences for anyone at any time of his lifetime.

So, achieving proper nutrition is very important and the ways of achieving it have great importance.

Hence, knowing what is a balanced diet and how to achieve it will be a great topic of importance as this is by far, one of the salient dietary hacks of all time.

What is a Balanced Diet?

For your diet to be a healthy one, you need to take all the nutrients in adequate amounts so your body will not have any deficiency for that nutrient. When you eat a certain food, it may have some of the essential nutrients that your body needs or it may contain a few.

Therefore, your diet needs a variety of food groups giving your body all the essential nutrient components in adequate amounts.

Simply, this is the definition of a balanced diet.

What are the Components of a Balanced Diet?

There are 7 essential components of a balanced diet. They are Carbohydrates, Proteins, Fats, Vitamins, Minerals, Fiber, and Water.

Each of these components does a vital part in body functions so you must include all of these in your diet in *adequate amounts*. Remember, too little is bad, and too much is also bad. That's why it is called a balanced diet!

Carbohydrates

Carbohydrates come into our bodies from starchy foods. They are abundant in cereals like rice, maize, wheat, etc., and some other starchy vegetables like potatoes, corn, etc. Once taken into our body, carbs are digested and converted into glucose.

This glucose is the main source of energy that the human brain and other organs consume to do their day-to-day functions. One gram of carbs can give your body 4 Calories of energy. If taken excess, your body will convert this glucose into fat and they will be deposited in fat stores.

Processed vs Unprocessed Grains,

Another important point to emphasize is that consuming unprocessed grains can not only give you carbs but also other nutrients like dietary fiber, vitamins, minerals, and phytonutrients.

Conversely, processing will reduce the amount of these other nutrients in the food reducing its nutritional value.

On the other hand, these processed grains can increase triglyceride levels in your blood while reducing beneficial HDL cholesterol levels. This is also not helpful to your body.

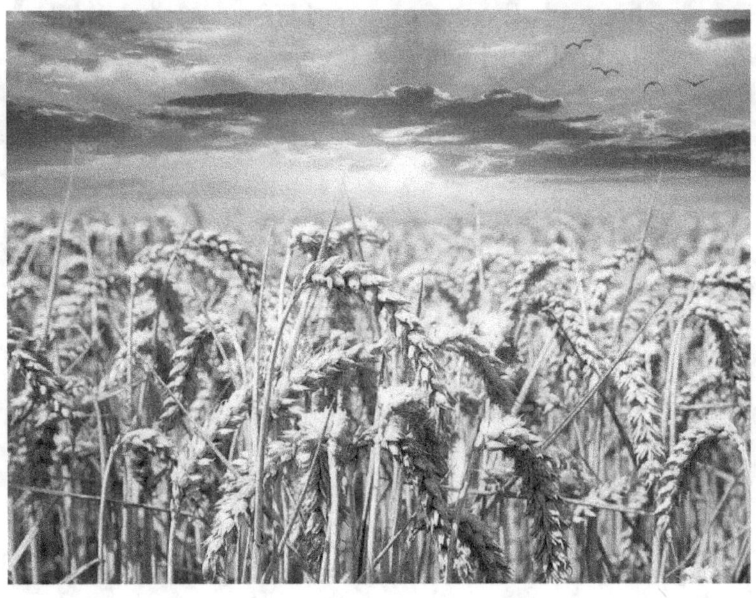

Hence, consuming white rice or white flour, etc. has less nutritional value when compared to the use of red rice or foods made with whole grains when used with fruits and vegetables.

Glycemic Index,

Similarly, there is a concept called the Glycemic index. Glycemic index refers to a value between 0 to 100 wherein it tells you how quickly your body digests carbs and how quickly glucose enters your bloodstream.

So, foods with a high glycemic index rapidly digest in the body and then absorbed. As a result, they increase your blood glucose levels quickly.

On the other hand, foods with a low glycemic index slowly increase your blood glucose levels. Thus, low glycemic index foods do not put your pancreas under great pressure to secrete large loads of insulin to drive away glucose into the cells.

Therefore, consuming a low glycemic index diet is very important in many ways to prevent diseases like diabetes.

The take-home message is that carbs are very important to provide fuel to your body and it helps the growth of your body, but excess use is also not good as it can lead you to diseases like diabetes. So, try to include low glycemic index foods in your balanced diet.

Proteins

Proteins are the main component of all the organ structures in the body. Besides, all the enzymes that potentiate all the chemical reactions in the body are proteins. Thus, proteins are very important so your balanced diet must include a rich supply of proteins.

When you take proteins, your digestive tract will digest them and form amino acids and absorb them into your body. Your body can make certain amino acids while you need to take some from outside. These are the essential amino acids. A well-balanced diet must contain all essential amino acids as you can't synthesize them in your body. Similarly, one gram of protein provides 4 calories of energy to your body.

You can add proteins to your balanced diet from plants and meat derivatives.

Plant proteins containing foods like beans, nuts, seeds, legumes, etc. are healthy food choices. Research says that consuming these will reduce the risk of getting cardiovascular diseases in later life.

Similarly, animal-based foods like meat, eggs, fish, etc. also contain good protein content but these foods will not reduce the risk of getting cardiovascular disease risk as these also contain high amounts of fats and other nutrients in excess amounts.

Dietary Fat

Traditionally, some people believed fats are bad as they increase cholesterol levels in the blood. But this is the wrong message. There is more to it.

Fats are indeed bad for the people who consume man-made hydrogenated oils that contain **trans fats**. Because these trans fats increase the harmful LDL (Low-density Lipoprotein) cholesterol level in your blood at the same time reducing your protective HDL (High-density Lipoprotein) cholesterol levels. Thus, trans fats increase the risk of cardiovascular diseases.

On the other hand, **Saturated fats** in the diet will increase both LDL and HDL cholesterol levels in your blood. So, you should consume saturated fats in moderate amounts and if taken excessively they can increase the risk of cardiovascular diseases as well. Saturated fats are abundant in Red meat, full cream milk, cheese, etc. You should eat these foods in moderate amounts in your balanced diet.

Monounsaturated and **polyunsaturated** fats are healthy fats. They come from sources like fish, seeds, nuts, whole grain, etc. As you can see, you can consume these fats mainly from a plant-based diet. Most importantly, there is a class of these fats called Omega 3 fats which comes from fish origin, has a wide array of health benefits.

Thus, if someone says fats are bad, that is a wrong statement. Therefore, unsaturated fats are an essential component of your balanced diet.

Vitamins and Minerals

Vitamins and Minerals are also very important components of a balanced diet. These act as antioxidants that help to protect your cells from free radical damage. Free radicals are the compounds that are formed due to the chemical reactions of the body and they are responsible for cell aging. Thus, these antioxidants in a balanced diet will keep you young!

Other than that, Vitamin A, B, C, D, E, and K acts as important co-factors in the essential body reactions, and also they are essential to improve your immunity as well. You can easily include vitamins in your balanced diet by adding fruits and vegetables. But keep in mind that it is beneficial if you can eat them fresh without much processing as excess processing can reduce their nutritional value.

Similarly, Minerals like Calcium are important for the growth and maintenance of your bones and teeth. Other minerals like Sodium, Potassium are important in maintaining neurological functions of the body. So, these are prime components of your balanced diet.

Dietary Fiber

Dietary fiber also a major component in a balanced diet. It helps your body in many ways. There are two parts of fiber. Firstly, **Soluble fiber**, as the name implies, is soluble in water. They lower your LDL cholesterol levels. They are abundant in foods like oats, beans, peas, fruits, etc.

Secondly, **Insoluble fiber**, which is not soluble in water so they pass down the digestive tract as intact compounds. They play a major role in stool formation thus preventing you from getting bowel problems like hemorrhoids etc. Insoluble fibers are abundant in whole grains, nuts, fruits, etc.

Water

Water is by far one of the essential components of a balanced diet. About 60 percent of our body weight is water. When the body is deprived of water, it can give very dangerous consequences. Water acts as a solvent for body chemicals and also it distributes heat throughout the body. The Health benefits of water should be a separate subject that we should know of.

The human body loses water via sweat, urine, feces, and respiratory passage. Other than that, the amount of loss of water from the body is dependent on physical activity, age, sex, etc. Therefore, we should replace water to keep our body functions intact.

How should we include water in our balanced diet?

Mostly, the food we take has water in it and they get absorbed into your body.

But as a rule, a person with 70 kg of body weight should take about 2.5 liters of water per day. If you take more water, the excess will be excreted in urine and so forth and it will not do any harm unless you are suffering from certain diseases like heart failure, kidney disease, etc.

Conversely, if you take less amount of water, it can lead to dehydration leading to very dangerous consequences.

How to take a Balanced Diet? – A Balanced Diet Plan

To answer the question of how to take a balanced diet, you should know the concept of the food pyramid. The food pyramid is a graphical representation or a guide to educate you what are the groups of foods you should be eating in what quantities to have a balanced diet, hence to have a healthy diet and lifestyle.

The food pyramid allows you to have a variety of food in moderation at the same time allowing you to enjoy different flavors, textures, colors, and odors, etc. in your food without counting calories. Ultimately, you will end up eating different groups of food in recommended quantities making a healthy diet.

The next chapter of this book explains everything about the food pyramid and the groups of foods that you should eat for a healthy life.

In short, you should try to eat more from the shelves that are near the base of the food pyramid. Conversely, you should restrict the number of servings from the topmost shelves of the food pyramid. That is to say, eat more fruits and vegetables. Similarly, consume unprocessed whole grains as much as possible.

Eat meat items and low-fat milk products in moderate amounts while eating pulses, dark green leaves adequately. Do not consume salt and sugars daily.

This is the main balanced diet plan that any individual should follow.

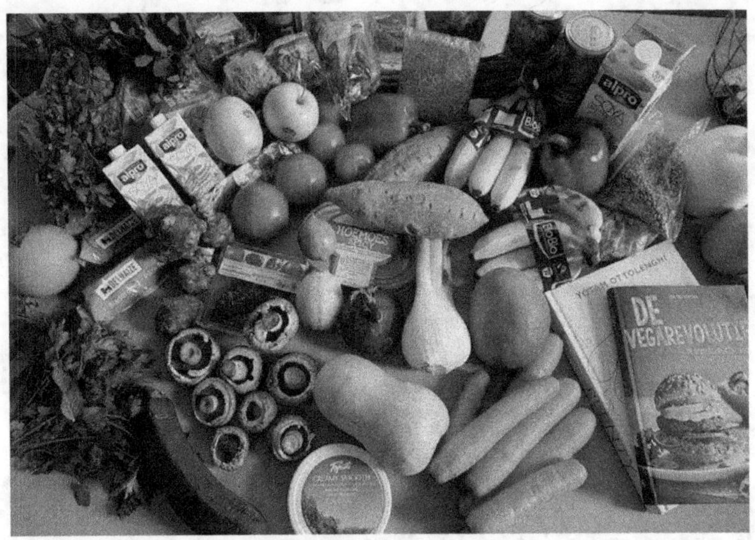

Always try to eat some foods from each shelf of the food pyramid per meal.

But this may be difficult so at least you can eat a variety of foods throughout the day maintaining that balance rather than eating a large quantity from a group of food from one shelf.

What are the Benefits of a Balanced Diet?

A Balanced Diet Helps to achieve Weight Loss

The main drawback of modern weight-loss diets is that you can't apply them to a whole society but just an individual only.

Although indeed, any single diet may not be suitable for everyone, a good diet should give the user a wide array of food choices with only a few restrictions. At the same time, it should give the user adequate nutrition that he needs while reducing the weight.

A balanced diet is a great example of this kind of diet. It gives you a lot of food choices while providing you with the intended nutrients.

Maintaining low glycemic index foods and avoiding refined grains and cutting down trans fats and reducing saturated fats will reduce your weight while giving you adequate nutrients.

Unlike other specific diets, anyone can consume a balanced diet quite easily.

It Reduces the Risk of Non-Communicable Diseases

As we discussed above, consuming a balanced diet ensures that you take an adequate amount of carbohydrates, proteins, and unsaturated fats.

This lets you cut down the refined grains from your diet adhering to a low glycemic index diet. Similarly, this lets you take fewer amounts of saturated fats with caution and avoid trans fats as much as possible.

A balanced diet ensures the increase of your good HDL cholesterol while reducing bad LDL cholesterol.

All of these will reduce the risk of cardiovascular diseases. And also, the consumption of low glycemic index foods will ensure your good health preventing you from getting diabetes. So, a balanced diet can keep you away from non-communicable diseases.

Effect on Pregnancy and Fertility

Research says that maintaining a balanced diet can cure women's ovarian infertility.

That is by cutting down trans fats while using more unsaturated fats in your diet, consuming whole grains rather than using refined grains, taking more plant-based proteins while reducing saturated fats coming from animals, cutting down sugary drinks and foods, and taking adequate amounts of foods containing iron, folate, and vitamins.

These are proven ways that can cure women's ovarian infertility by modern research.

Similarly, these dietary habits with the use of omega 3 fat usage in pregnancy can prevent neurological defects in the fetuses too.

This is a great benefit of a balanced diet for women and their babies to ensure good health in both mother and her baby.

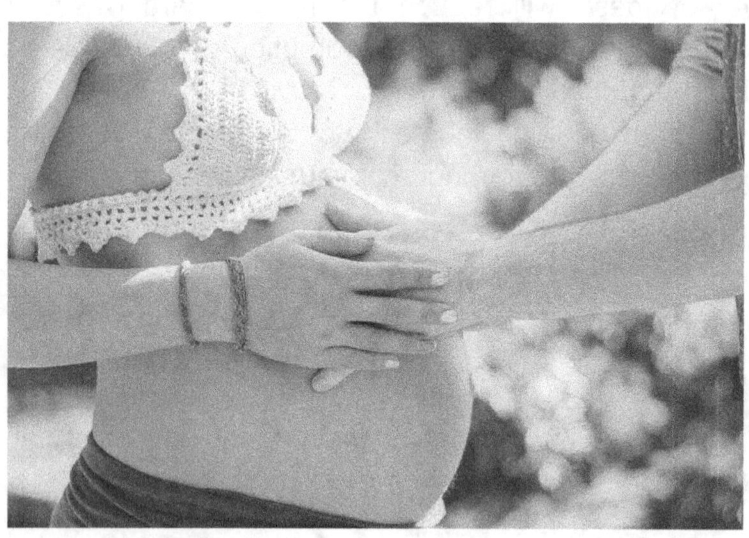

It Boosts the Immune System

Vitamins and minerals are important as antioxidants preventing free radical damage to your cells. And also, they are important co-factors in many biochemical reactions in the body.

Likewise, they boost your immune system providing safety from outside pathogenic organisms too.

A balanced diet ensures you take adequate amounts of fruits and vegetables leading to a rich supply of vitamins and minerals in your body boosting your immunity.

Prevents Illnesses due to Dietary Deficiencies

A wide array of illnesses can occur if you don't take certain nutrients like vitamins, trace elements, etc.

Iron deficiency, Vitamin B12 deficiency, Folate deficiency, Individual vitamin deficiencies are a few of them.

When you are taking a balanced diet, you are taking each nutrient in adequate amounts so you will not face these illnesses that are due to the dietary deficiency of that particular nutrient.

Balanced Diet for a Vegan

A balanced diet for a vegetarian is also an important topic.

As you know, the main drawback of a vegan diet is that since they lack the animal protein component that comes from shelf four of the food pyramid.

So, they are more prone to get nutritional deficiencies like iron deficiency, Vitamin B12 deficiency, and protein deficiency.

Therefore, all vegans must include plenty of pulses, seeds, and nuts in their diet.
Similarly, you should eat cereals, fruits, and vegetables, and dark green leaves as much as possible to ensure the intake of these nutrients.

Likewise, you need a good intake of low-fat milk products to ensure good protein intake to help in the growth and maintenance of the body.

A vegan diet is one of the enjoyable and nutritionally sound diets if you plan it carefully.

In Conclusion,

To sum up, although it is true that any single diet may not be suitable for everyone, a balanced diet gives the user a wide array of food choices with only a few restrictions.

At the same time, it gives the user adequate nutrition that he needs for the maintenance of healthy body functions.

Maintaining a balanced diet by cutting down trans fats while using more unsaturated fats, consuming whole grain rather than using refined grains, taking more plant-based proteins while reducing saturated fats coming from animals, cutting down sugary drinks and foods, and taking adequate amounts of foods containing iron, folate and vitamins can cure a wide array of non-communicable diseases and women's infertility problems.

With these health facts, needless to say, that consuming a balanced diet is one of the greatest dietary hacks that you need to know for a healthy life!

Chapter 2.

What is the Food Pyramid: Eat these Foods Now for a Healthy Life!

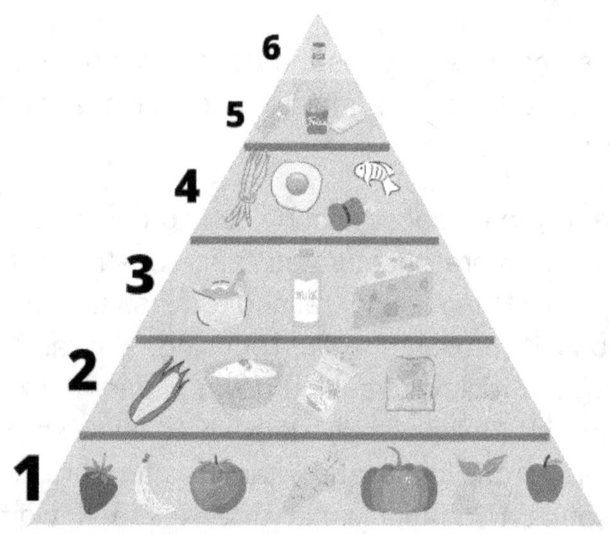

There is a common saying that "You are what you eat".

It is far more relevant to these times as the prevalence of cancer and other non-communicable diseases like diabetes, stroke, etc. are rising day by day.

Research says that these illnesses have a strong association with your diet. Thus, consuming a diet with *healthy groups of food* in *adequate amounts* will permit a healthy life.

This is the importance of knowing what is the food pyramid!

What is the Food Pyramid?

The food pyramid is a graphical representation or a guide to educate you what are the groups of food you should be eating in what quantities to have a balanced diet, hence to have a healthy diet and lifestyle.

Traditionally, the old food pyramid had 4 shelves but the U.S. Department of Agriculture (USDA) had altered the food pyramid in 2005 to a new pyramid with 5 main shelves and another topmost shelf which is separated from the main pyramid.

They considered all the up-to-date knowledge and scientific evidence while preparing this new food pyramid.

And for the rest of this article, we will be considering this new food pyramid as a guide to what you should eat to be healthy!

What is the Importance of the Food Pyramid?

Eating is one of the greatest joys of life. But if you eat the same kind of food every day, you may have experienced that it doesn't give you the enjoyment that you are expecting from this endeavor.

However, imagine changing the amount of food you eat and changing the variety of food with each meal.

The food pyramid allows you to have a variety of food in moderation at the same time allowing you to enjoy different flavors, textures, colors, and odors, etc. in your food without counting calories.

Ultimately, you will end up eating different groups of food in recommended quantities making a healthy diet.

What are the Groups of Food on different Shelves in the Food Pyramid?

Before we jump into different food groups, it is very important to verify the serving size of each meal from each shelf of the food pyramid.

The truth is that the number of servings per day depends on age, sex, level of activity, body size, whether suffering from illnesses, and the geographic region of the person in the world.

For instance, if you are having a good physical activity in your workplace or an athlete etc. the number of servings you need will be different from a person who is an inactive office worker.

Similarly, the number of servings per day for a person from a tropical country will differ from for a person from a temperate country.

Therefore, if you want to measure the exact serving size, you have to consult your local area nutritionist.

We will be guiding you to have an idea of what to eat and what not to eat!

Most importantly, you can make variations in your diet even within the same food group by changing the color, taste, and way of preparation.

For example, when you are taking vegetables, you can prepare salads, or even eat them fresh.

Likewise, you can add different colors to your food plate by choosing different vegetables.

Shelf one – The base of the pyramid

This shelf contains all the fruits and vegetables. These are very important as they contain different classes of antioxidants and vitamins so that they will keep you away from diseases.

Shelf two – the one above to the base

This shelf contains all starchy food that contains carbohydrates. Cereals, rice, corn, and preparations from the wheat flour like bread, etc.

These are very important as they provide you energy to carry out your day-to-day activities.

Shelf three

This shelf contains milk preparations. Milk, yogurt, curd, cheese are the most popular items.
These foods are important in the growth and maintenance of your bone health as they consist of micronutrients like Calcium.

Thus, they are very important to prevent you get disease conditions like Osteoporosis, etc.

Try to consume low-fat milk preparations and you can opt to eat or drink more milk and yogurt when compared to cheese.

Shelf four

This shelf contains fish, meat, pulses, and eggs. These are protein products and important in the growth of your body.

Lean meat, eggs, non-oily Fish are good choices whereas salty preparations like bacon, ham, sausages are better used in moderation. Pulses like chickpeas, green gram, etc. are healthy food choices.

Shelf five

This is the top shelf within the new food pyramid. This shelf contains oils, fat, and spreads.

These fats are important in providing energy that helps in bodily functions.

Try to use mono or polyunsaturated oils or spreads as much as possible. Olive oil, coconut oil, sunflower oil are good choices.

Moreover, try to use the minimum amount of oil for food preparation while cooking, baking, deep-frying, etc.

Shelf six – The topmost shelf that is separated from the new food pyramid

This shelf contains foods that are high in fat, sugar, and salt. You should not consume these daily. But using very small amounts once or twice a week may not do any harm.

Other Important Considerations

Always try to eat some foods from each shelf of the food pyramid per meal. But this may be difficult so at least you can eat a variety of foods throughout the day maintaining that balance rather than eating a large quantity from a group of food from one shelf.

This will help you ensure that your diet consists of all the nutrients in adequate amounts.

Should I take Supplements?

Yes. But some researchers say that these nutrients have interactions with each other within your body.

For instance, high-dose iron supplements can cause your body to not absorb as much zinc as you may need.

Likewise, not getting enough zinc can cause problems with some key functions of the immune system. On the other hand, too much zinc can interfere with copper absorption.

Thus, it is very important to gain all these nutrients with your daily portion of a balanced diet.

With an understanding of what is the food pyramid and the groups of food that you should eat, you can fulfill this easily.

However, you may need to consult a professional if you want to use an additional supplement in this regard.

Vegan's Food Pyramid

By now you may be wondering if you are a vegan, what is the food pyramid that you should be using to achieve a healthy diet. That is simple.

As we have discussed in the first chapter, the main drawback of a vegan diet is that since they lack the animal protein component that comes from shelf four.

So, they are more prone to get nutritional deficiencies like iron deficiency, Vitamin B12 deficiency, and protein deficiency.

Therefore, all vegans must include plenty of pulses, seeds, and nuts in their diet.

Similarly, you should eat cereals, fruits, and vegetables, and dark green leaves as much as possible to ensure the intake of these nutrients.

Likewise, you need a good intake of milk products to ensure good protein intake to help in the growth and maintenance of the body.

In Conclusion,

To sum up, there are 6 shelves in the new food pyramid while the topmost shelf is separated from the rest.

You should try to eat more from the shelves that are near the base of the food pyramid. Conversely, you should restrict the number of servings from the topmost shelves of the food pyramid.

Always try to eat some foods from each shelf of the food pyramid per meal.

But this may be difficult so at least you can eat a variety of foods throughout the day maintaining that balance rather than eating a large quantity from a group of food from one shelf.

The food pyramid allows you to have a variety of food in moderation at the same time allowing you to enjoy different flavors, textures, colors, and odors, etc. in your food without counting calories.

Ultimately, you will end up eating different groups of food in recommended quantities making a healthy diet.

Chapter 3.

Benefits of Low Glycemic Index Diet for Healthy Life!

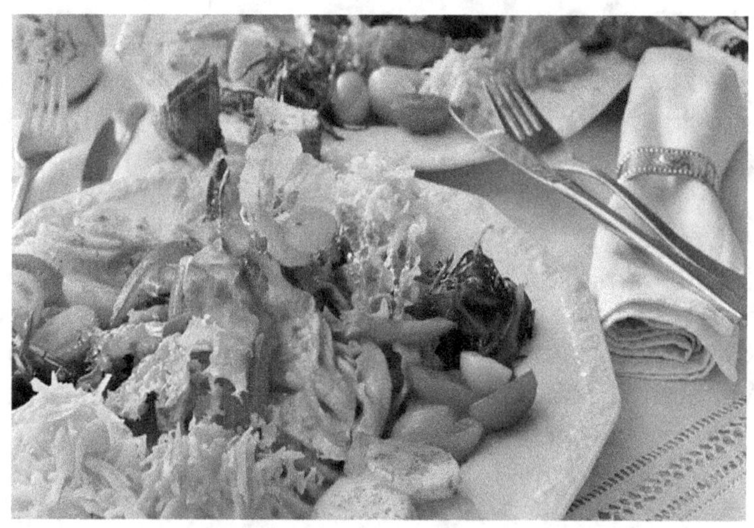

What is the Glycemic Index (GI)?

There are lots of benefits of consuming a low glycemic index diet.

The glycemic index (GI) is a ranking of carbohydrates on a scale from 0 to 100. This is based on how each of the food categories raises blood sugar levels after eating.

In other words, the glycemic index is a value assigned to food based on how slowly or how quickly they increase sugar levels in the blood.

To clarify, when you eat or drink something with carbohydrates, your body breaks down the sugars and starches into a type of simple sugar. This is called glucose which is the main source of energy for cells in your body.

Then afterward, your pancreas secretes the hormone insulin. The action of insulin is to drive the absorbed glucose from your digestive tract into the cells of the body.

Different types of carbohydrate foods have different properties. In which how quickly your body digests them and how quickly glucose enters your bloodstream.

So, food with a high glycemic index rapidly digests in the body and is then absorbed. As a result, they increase your blood glucose levels quickly.

On the other hand, food with a low glycemic index slowly increases your blood glucose levels. Thus, low glycemic index food does not put your pancreas under great pressure to secrete large loads of insulin to drive away glucose into the cells.

Hence, this is beneficial to your body as we all know that "high blood sugar" or blood glucose levels above normal are toxic and can cause blindness, kidney failure, increase heart attacks, and other problems like diabetic foot, etc.

Thus, consuming a low glycemic index diet is a part of a balanced diet too.

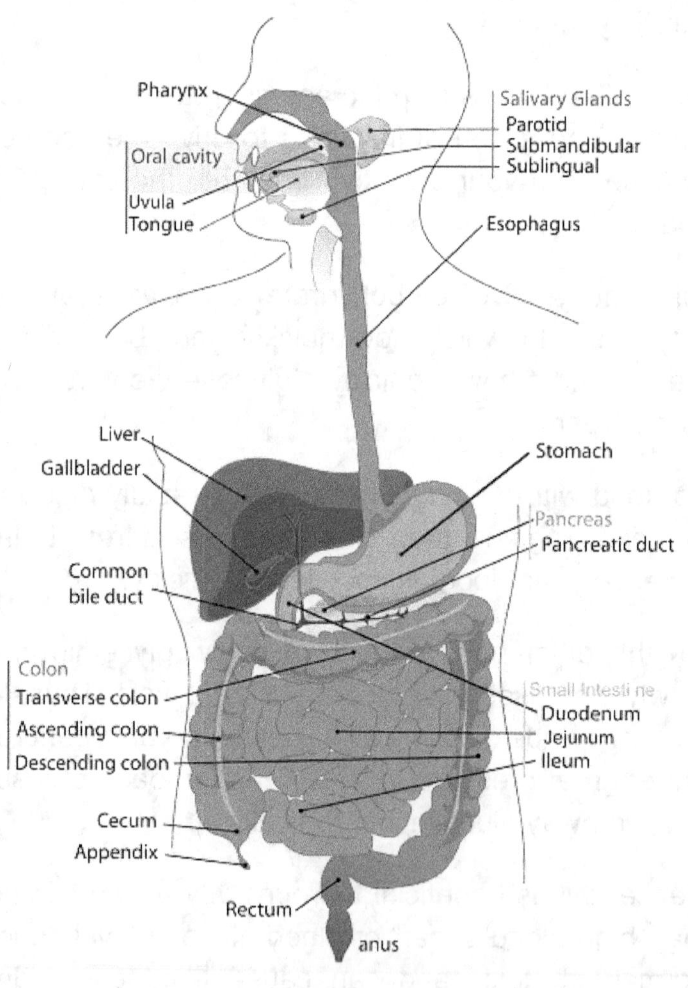

How to know What Food has a Low Glycemic Index?

- ***The low glycemic index (GI of 55 or less):***
  - Most fruits and vegetables, beans, chickpeas, minimally processed grains, pasta, low-fat dairy food, dates, and nuts.

- ***The moderate glycemic index (GI 56 to 69):***
  - White and sweet potatoes, corn, white rice, couscous, breakfast cereals such as Cream of Wheat and Mini-Wheats.

- ***The high glycemic index (GI of 70 or higher):***
  - White bread, rice cakes, most crackers, bagels, cakes, doughnuts, croissants, most packaged breakfast cereals.

By analyzing this, you can understand it is better to consume foods from the low GI category instead of those in the high GI category.

And you can go easy on those in between.

Health Benefits of Consuming Low Glycemic Index Diet

It Helps to Control Diabetes

Following extensive research, all major diabetes organizations around the world recommend consuming a low GI diet in the management of diabetes as part of the nutritional management of the condition.

Furthermore, researchers are suggesting that it is the most appropriate dietary intervention for pregnant mothers with diabetes as well.

Helps to Control High Cholesterol Levels in Blood

Researchers have found out that combining a low GI diet with high fiber content would reduce the low-density lipoprotein cholesterols. These are the bad cholesterols.

In addition to this, consuming low to moderate GI food like fresh fruits, vegetables, and whole grains would increase the fiber amount in your diet as well.

Promotes Weight Loss and Appetite Control

Some studies show that consuming a low GI diet may promote weight loss and help to maintain lost weight.

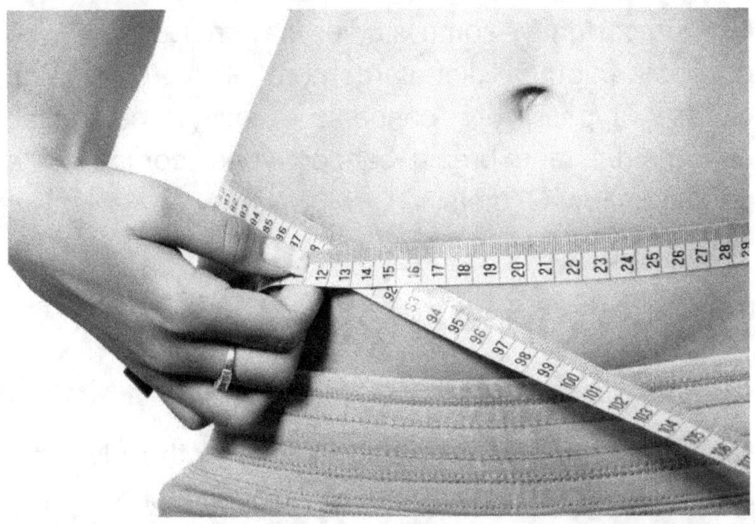

Similarly, studies show more weight gain by consuming diets with a high GI such as eating refined grains, starches, and sugars.

Concerning that, high-GI food causes a rapid increase in blood glucose, a rapid insulin response. Subsequently, this would lead to a rapid return to feeling hungry.

By contrast, Low-GI food would delay feelings of hunger as they maintain a steady state of blood glucose level.

May Reduce the Risk of Cancer

Most importantly, some studies say that people who consume high-GI diets are more likely to develop certain types of cancers. Mostly colorectal, endometrial, and breast cancer types, compared to people on low-GI diets.

Other Considerations

However, there are some limitations in the glycemic index values. The most important drawback is that it doesn't reflect the quantity that you should consume a particular food.

Some fruits like watermelon have a high GI value but they have a few digestible carbohydrates in one serving. In other words, you have to eat a lot of watermelons to significantly raise your blood glucose level.

To address this problem, researchers have developed the idea of **glycemic load (GL)**. Which is a numerical value that indicates the change in blood glucose levels when you eat a typical serving of a particular food.

So, although some food with high GI value might fall into the healthy food category depending on the amount you consume.

GL value also falls into three categories,

- **Low:** 10 or less
- **Medium:** 11–19
- **High:** 20 or more

If you can consume foods that fall into the low GL category, those would be the safest and healthiest type of food to eat.

However, GI is still the most important factor to consider when following the low-GI diet. Moreover, the Glycemic Index Foundation, an Australian organization raising awareness about the low-GI diet, recommends that people also monitor their GL.

You can use the database of the University of Sydney, Australia to see these values for certain foods. They researched glycemic index food to find the GI and GL values of common food.

Another pitfall of GI value is that it tells us nothing about other nutritional information other than carbohydrates.

Some foods, like whole milk, have a low GI value but contains a high amount of fat content. Thus, it would not be a good choice if you are planning on a weight loss regime.

In Conclusion,

To sum up, picking good sources of carbohydrates can help you control your blood sugar and your weight.

The benefits of consuming a low glycemic index diet can help prevent a host of chronic conditions. Especially diabetes and hypercholesterolemia but it can also promote weight loss and ward off various cancers as well.

Chapter 4.

Amazing Health Benefits of Consuming Omega 3 Fatty Acids in Diet

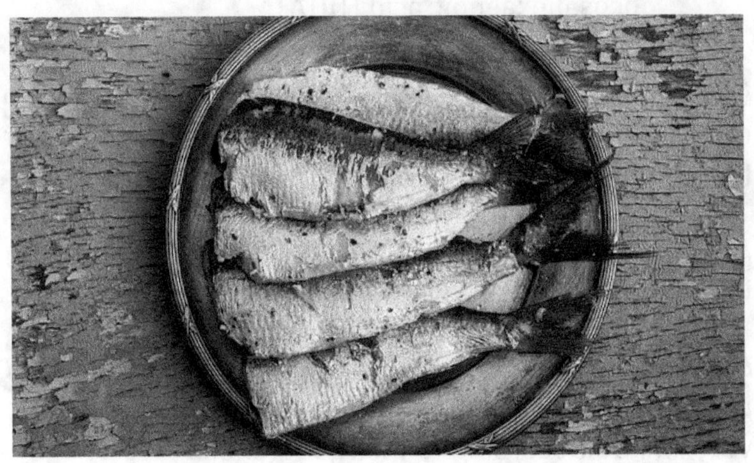

What are Omega 3 Fatty Acids?

Consuming Omega 3 fatty acids in the diet is very important as they give you tons of health benefits.

Omega 3 fatty acids are a type of polyunsaturated fatty acids consists of long chains of carbon atoms with a carboxyl group at one end of the chain and a methyl group at the other.

This is one of the important components that you should include in your balanced diet.

There are several different omega 3s that exist, but the majority of scientific research focuses on three of them;

- alpha-linolenic acid (ALA)
- eicosapentaenoic acid (EPA)
- docosahexaenoic acid (DHA)

(Certainly, if you are not really into chemistry, you do not have to remember these names. Just remember them as Omega 3s!)

ALA is considered an essential fatty acid, meaning that it must be obtained from the diet.

ALA can be converted into EPA and then to DHA, but the conversion which occurs primarily in the liver is very limited according to the researches.

Therefore, consuming EPA and DHA directly from food or dietary supplements is the only practical way to increase levels of these fatty acids in the body.

ALA is rich in plant oils, such as flaxseed, soybean, and canola oils.

DHA and EPA are present in fish, fish oils, and krill oils, but originally microalgae which is a kind of seaweed produce these not by the fish. When fish consume phytoplankton that consumed microalgae, they accumulate the omega-3s in their tissues.

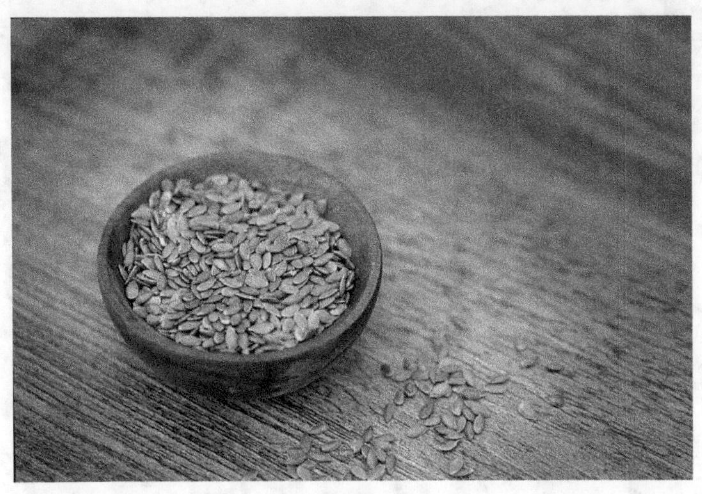

Flax seeds are a plant-based source of omega 3 fatty acids

Important Benefits of Omega 3 Fatty Acids in the Diet

As Components of Organ Structures in the Body

Omega 3s play important roles in the body as components of the phospholipids that form the structures of cell membranes.

DHA, in particular, is especially high in the retina of the eye, brain, and sperm.

Besides, omega 3s provide energy for the body and form signaling molecules hence have wide-ranging functions in the body's cardiovascular, pulmonary, immune, and endocrine systems.

They Lower the Risk of getting Cardiovascular Disease

Many studies have assessed the effects of omega 3s on high blood pressure and elevated blood lipid levels etc.

One of those studies had found low rates of heart attacks and other heart-related diseases among Greenland Inuit and other fish-eating populations, such as the Japanese.

Aids in Neuro-Development and Infant Health

Lots of studies have examined the effects of mothers' seafood and omega 3 intakes on infant birth weight, length of pregnancy, healthy eyesight and brain development, and other infant health outcomes.

Mainly, DHA is important for fetal growth and development. The accumulation of DHA in the retina of the eye is completed by birth, whereas accumulation in the brain continues throughout the first 2 years after birth.

However, seafood contains varying levels of mercury and other toxins. These include mackerel, wild swordfish, tilefish, and sharks. But, fish like wild trout and wild salmon, sardines are safer.

Helps to Prevent Cancer

Researchers have found that higher intakes of omega 3s from either foods or supplements might reduce the risk of certain cancers like breast cancer, colorectal cancer, etc.

This is probably a result of their anti-inflammatory effects and the potential to inhibit cell growth factors.

Helps to have Healthy Eyes

DHA is a major structural component of your eye's retina. Thus, it may help prevent visual impairment and blindness.

Will reduce the risk of dry eye disease and relieve its symptoms because of their anti-inflammatory activity and many patients take them in addition to the treatment like artificial tears and other medications.

Helps you Fight Auto-Immune Diseases

In autoimmune diseases what happens is your immune system mistakes healthy cells for foreign cells and starts attacking them.

Studies show that getting enough omega 3s during your first year of life is linked to a reduced risk of many autoimmune diseases including type-1 diabetes and multiple sclerosis etc.

Omega-3s also help treat lupus, rheumatoid arthritis, ulcerative colitis, Crohn's disease, and psoriasis.

Helps you Fight Depression

Some researchers have found that cultures that eat food with high levels of omega-3s have lower levels of depression.

Furthermore, studies have shown that when people with depression or anxiety start taking omega-3 supplements their symptoms improve.

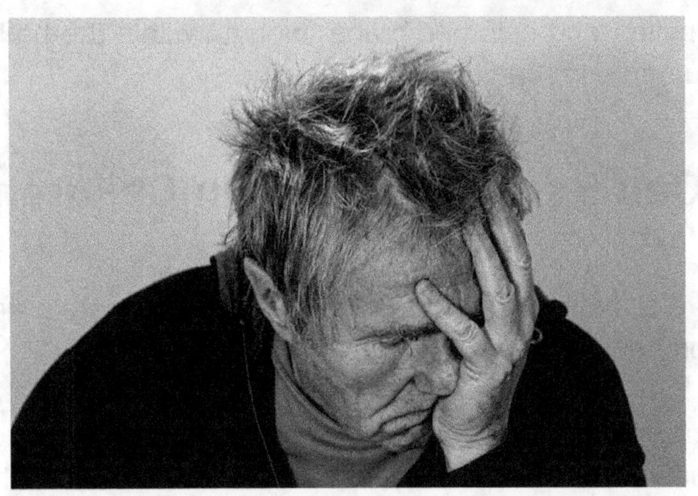

One of the important benefits of consuming Omega 3 Fatty Acids in your diet is that it helps you fight depression

Can Help you in Alzheimer's Disease, Dementia, and Maintaining Cognitive Function

Some studies suggest that diets high in omega 3s are associated with a reduced risk of cognitive decline, Alzheimer's disease, and dementia because DHA is an essential component of the cellular membrane in the brain.

Researchers think that omega 3s might protect cognitive function by helping to maintain neuronal function and cell membrane integrity within the brain. But more research should be done.

Can Reduce Asthma in Children

A diet high in omega 3s lowers inflammation a key component in asthma.

But more studies are needed to show if fish oil supplements improve your lung function or cut the amount of medication a person with asthma needs to control the condition.

Can Improve your Skin Health

DHA is a structural component of your skin. That is to say, it is responsible for the health of cell membranes which make up a large part of your skin.
A healthy cell membrane results in soft, moist, supple, and wrinkle-free skin.

Consuming high amounts of Omega 3s also helps to manage oil production and hydration of your skin reducing the risk of acne and also reducing premature aging of your skin.

Should I take Fish oil Supplements?

The simple answer is *Yes*.

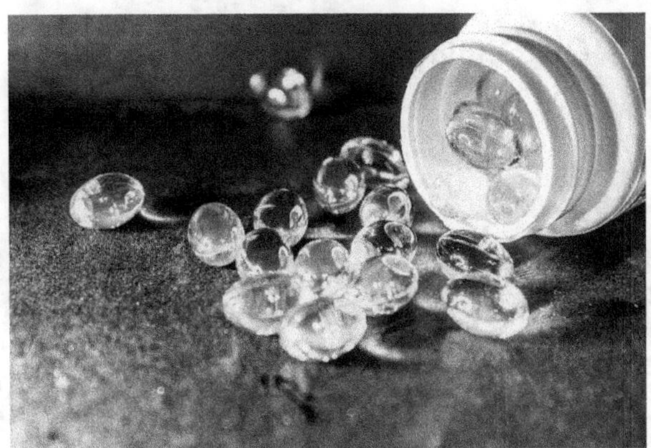

Fish oil supplement capsules

Fish oil, algae oil has DHA and may be a good option for people who don't eat fish. The most common side effects of fish oil are indigestion and gas. Getting a supplement with a coating might help.

However, talk to your doctor about taking a supplement first. He or she may have specific recommendations or warnings depending on your health and the other medicines you take.

For example, Omega 3 supplements can make bleeding more likely. If you have a bleeding condition or taking medicines that could increase bleeding like clopidogrel, warfarin, and some NSAIDs, etc. talk to your doctor before using any omega 3 supplements.

In Conclusion,

To sum up, Consuming Omega 3 fatty acids in your diet will give you tons of health benefits.

Adding fish oil supplements can augment those benefits. Always talk to your doctor before taking any supplements.

Chapter 5.

Great Health Benefits of Coconut Water that will Blow your Mind Away!

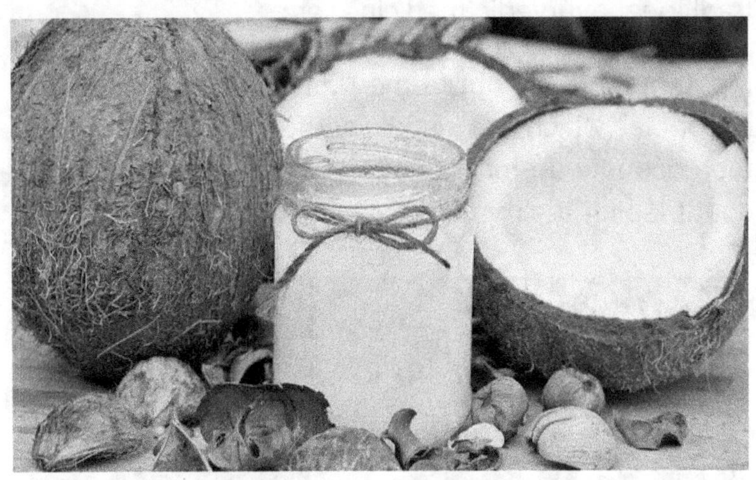

What are Coconuts?

Coconuts are botanically known as *cocos nucifera*. It is a famous fruit readily available in the tropics. It is very famous not only for the health benefits of coconut water inside but also for its other uses as well.

Certainly, various parts of coconut fruit are valuable to people in many ways. They use the trunk and leaves of this fruit to make constructing substances, for instance, roofing of the houses, etc.

Similarly, oil extracted from the fruit is an excellent component used in food processing while the husk of the fruit is processed to make carpets, ropes, mats, etc. In the same vein, coconut shells are used as charcoal and the root of the tree is widely used as traditional ayurvedic medicine, etc.

Most importantly, unlike the "king coconuts" or "yellow coconuts" which are used only for their water inside, the coconuts are precious to the people in the tropical countries for their various uses mentioned above.

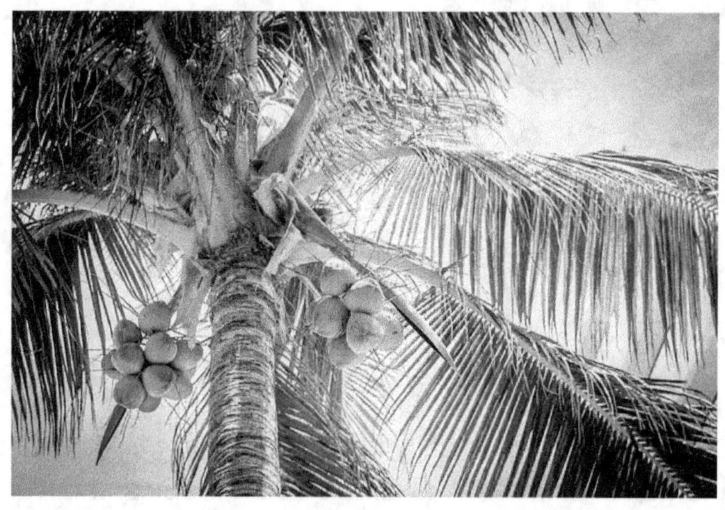

The coconut tree is a famous fruit in tropical countries

Depending on the age of the fruit, the taste of the water within and the uses of this fruit vary. Hence, the young green coconuts are most suitable for drinking purposes while the aged coconut fruits are used in processes like cooking, etc.

Amazing Health Benefits of Coconut Water

Rich in All Nutrients

Coconut water is a rich source of natural electrolytes, amino acids, vitamins, trace elements, and minerals, etc. Besides, it is low in sugar but has a pleasant sweet taste as well.

Other than these, it contains antioxidants and various bioactive enzymes which are important in various cellular functions in the body.

These will keep your body free from diseases and help generate energy for the body. At the same time, these compounds aid in digestion and improve the overall metabolism of the body as well.

It's a Great Natural Solution to Prevent Dehydration

It will naturally replenish the body's loss of electrolytes by sweating during exercise or any other type of exertion.
Subsequently, this will help prevent dehydration and fatigue.

Owing to these properties of coconut water it is a great solution for athletes to use as a natural sports drink for oral hydration.

Additionally, according to the researchers, coconut water is non-allergenic and readily accepted by the human body. Likewise, it has no harmful effects on the red blood cells too. Thus, it is an excellent rehydrating solution for all.

This is by far, one of the greatest health benefits of coconut water compared to commercial drinks in the market nowadays.

Good for a Healthy Heart

The research found that coconut water can reduce your blood pressure. Furthermore, it can reduce the harmful cholesterol levels in your body too.

Therefore, it can decrease the potential of forming clots in your blood vessels and promote a healthy heart and circulatory system.

Besides, some studies say that coconut water is good for your red blood cells and it can be a remedy to anemia as well.

Helps to Prevent Kidney Stones

Coconut water is a natural diuretic. That is to say, it increases your urinary output while diluting urine and flushes off the urinary tract. This aids to keep your urinary tract free from bacteria and viruses keeping you away from urinary tract infections.

On the other hand, substances in coconut water can prevent the formation of certain types of kidney stones. So, consuming coconut water in your diet promotes good healthy kidneys and urinary tract.

Helps to Control Sugar Level in Diabetics

Studies found that substances in coconut water can act on the receptor level of the insulin hormone which is responsible to reduce your sugar levels.

That is to say, it improves the function of insulin causing lowering effects on your sugar levels.

So, this is good news for diabetics. Unlike commercial hydrating solutions, you can consume coconut water without the fear of getting high sugars!

Promotes Good Immunity

Promoting good immune function is another one of the health benefits of coconut water.

Antimicrobial lipids and other compounds found in coconut water have antifungal, antimicrobial, and antiviral properties. Therefore, needless to say, that consuming coconut water boosts your immune function.

Moreover, coconut water can act on and prevent intestinal worms. Above all, it is effective in treating gastrointestinal diseases and useful in treating cholera too.

Further, it improves constipation as well as being effective in treating diarrhea in babies too.

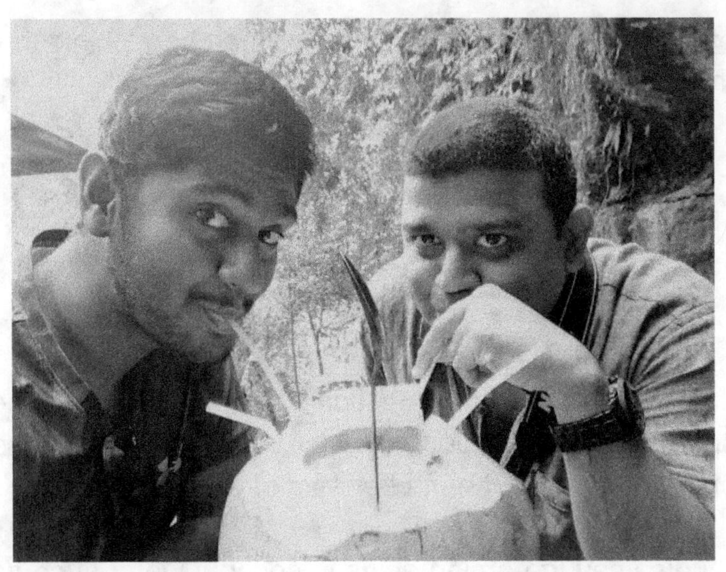

Enjoying coconut water from the fruit could be a great recreational activity when compared to the health benefits of coconut water!

It has Antioxidant Properties

In our human body when oxygen is metabolized, it creates unstable molecules called "oxygen free radicals". Above all, these steel electrons from other important molecules of the cells of the body. This is called an oxidative process. Therefore, these damages cell membranes, DNA molecules, cellular proteins, etc.

Antioxidants are the molecules that act on these oxygen-free radicals. They prevent and break harmful effects on the body. Further, researchers think that these antioxidants can prevent cancer as well.

Coconut water is a rich source of antioxidants!

It Boosts Fertility

If you are asking the question of how to increase the sperm count, it is good news for you! This topic is one of the other great health benefits of coconut water.

Studies say the amino acids in coconut water such as L-arginine can increase the sperm count in males and improves the motility of the sperm.

Similarly, some people believe their sperm taste better when they consume coconut water. This may be true as coconut water improves the quantity and quality of body fluids in the body so it should improve the quality and quantity of your sperm too.

Therefore, does coconut water increase your sperm volume? The answer is yes.

Moreover, substances in coconut water have beneficial effects on the sex hormones in both males and females. As a result of these, it is likely to increase fertility in people of the right age.

Beware!

However, some studies reported that people with certain diseases should alarm themselves while consuming excessive amounts of coconut water.

So, how much coconut water should I drink?

The answer is "it depends".

For instance, if you are suffering from diabetes, chronic renal impairment, and potassium retaining medication, there is a high risk of developing "hyperkalemia" which is a condition where you get excessive potassium levels in the blood if you consume too much. This is due to its high potassium content.

But don't worry.

If you are suffering from any of these diseases consult your doctor and take advice. With your doctor's advice, still you can consume and enjoy the benefits of this amazing natural product.

In Conclusion,

To sum up, there are a lot of health benefits of coconut water.

Certainly, since it is a natural product rich in all the nutrients and electrolytes it is an excellent rehydrating solution. It promotes a healthy heart, kidneys, and boosts immunity.

However, be cautious when you consume excessive amounts if you have certain diseases as it can overload your potassium levels in the body!

Although it's freely available in commercial preparations, needless to say, not only its benefits but also the pure enjoyment it gives when you consume it naturally from the fruit. Don't forget to enjoy this fruit on your next trip to the tropics!

Chapter 6.

Antioxidant Food for better Health and Long Life!

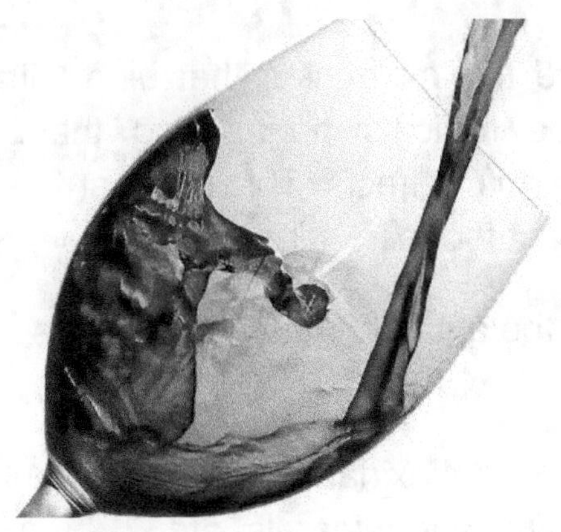

What is an Antioxidant Food?

Antioxidant foods are very important for better health.

Because in our human body when the oxygen is metabolized, it creates unstable molecules called "oxygen free radicals". Above all, these steel electrons from other important molecules of the cells of the body, and called an oxidative process. Therefore, these damages cell membranes, DNA molecules, cellular proteins, etc.

Most importantly, our body can cope with this damage to some extent. Nevertheless, if this oxidative stress is overloaded, the body is prone to get certain diseases like heart disease, liver disease, cancers and it will accelerate the aging process also.

This is when antioxidants come into play.

Certainly, they are the molecules that bind with the above oxygen-free radicals neutralizing them and preventing their harmful effects. This is by far the best benefit of antioxidant foods.

They can prevent the aging of all of your organs in the body.

Moreover, these antioxidants include nutrient antioxidants, vitamins, and minerals, etc.

Imagine having good healthy skin in your sixties and imagine having a healthy heart, lungs in your sixties. I think you understand the benefits of consuming antioxidant-rich foods.

Antioxidant-Rich Food Groups

Firstly, antioxidant-rich foods are fruits and vegetables. Other than that; nuts, wholegrain, fish, dark chocolates are rich in antioxidants too.

The following antioxidant food list will help you understand what are the groups of food that you should include in your balanced diet.

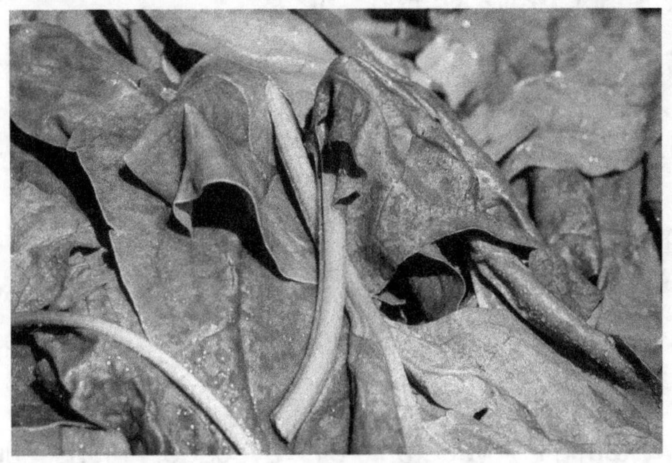

Spinach, green leaves are rich a source of antioxidants

Some Examples of Specific Antioxidant Types are;

1. Beta carotene – carrots, mangoes, pumpkins, spinach

2. Catechins – red wine, tea

3. Flavonoids - tea, green tea, red wine, onions, citrus fruits

4. Lutein – green leafy vegetables like spinach, corn

5. Lycopene – tomatoes, watermelon

6. Lignans – whole grains, bran, sesame seeds

7. Copper – milk, seafood, nuts

8. Indoles – broccoli, cauliflower, cabbage

9. Manganese – seafood, milk, nuts

10. Vitamin A – carrots, milk, egg yolk, sweet potatoes

11. Vitamin C – Oranges, kiwifruit, mangoes, strawberries

12. Vitamin E – vegetable oils, avocado, nuts, seeds

13. Zinc – seafood, milk, nuts

How Should I Take Antioxidants?

Is it worth taking antioxidant supplements or should I take them in my diet only? Let's find out!

Most importantly, a valuable point to emphasize is that if you take the above classes of compounds as supplements that it will not give the desired benefit.

That is because some compounds of certain classes of above interact with each other. Similarly, it will interfere with how your body absorbs those compounds.

For instance, high-dose iron supplements can cause your body to not absorb as much zinc as you may need.

Likewise, not getting enough zinc can cause problems with some key functions of the immune system. On the other hand, too much zinc can interfere with copper absorption.

Hence, if you take these from the natural way the more beneficial it is.

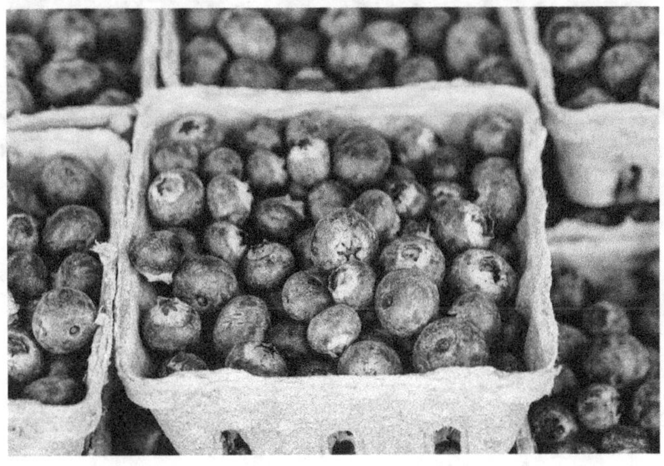

Blueberry – Another antioxidant-rich food

Measuring the Antioxidant Content in Foods

To clarify, Scientists use several tests to measure the antioxidant content of the food.

One of the best tests is the FRAP (ferric reducing ability of plasma) analysis. Further, it measures the antioxidant content of food by how well it can neutralize a specific free radical.

The higher the FRAP value, the more antioxidants the food contains. Thus, needless to say, you have to take more of the food that has a higher FRAP value.

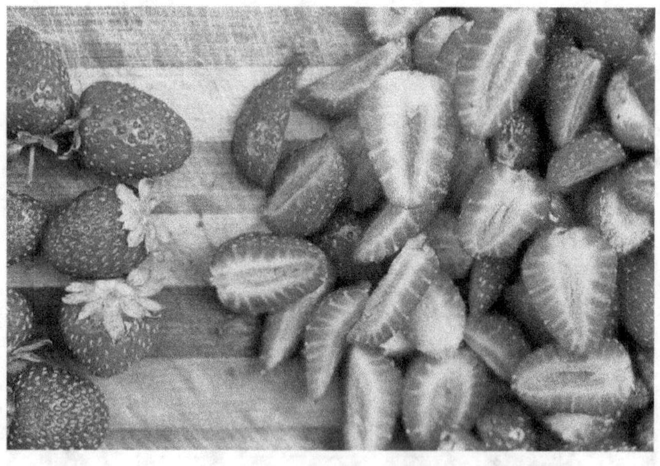

Strawberries – Another one of the antioxidant-rich fruits

In Conclusion,

To sum up, a diet with antioxidant containing foods is very important to have a healthy life not only for their nutritional value but also, they keep your cells young.

Chapter 7.

Value of Consuming Gluten-Free Diet for a Healthy Life!

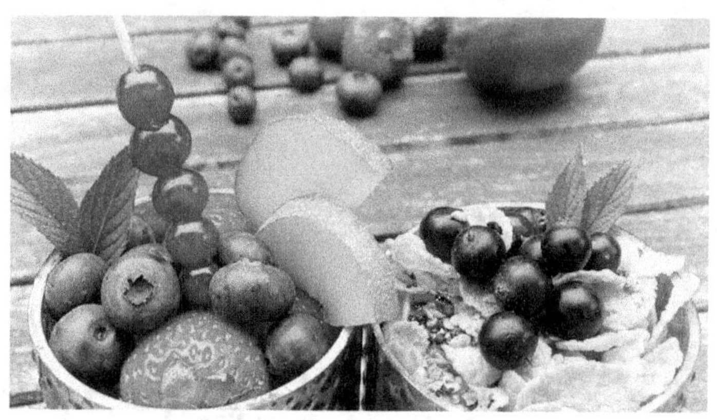

What is Gluten?

Consuming a gluten-free diet is very important if you are having gluten sensitivity. Gluten is protein-rich in food like barley, rye, oats, and wheat, etc. Certain people have high sensitivity to gluten as they consume food containing gluten.

Most importantly, these reactions will cause them to have different symptoms and signs and the severity of these symptoms varies from one person to another.

Likewise, it could be a small allergic reaction or heartburn that most people would ignore whereas it is called celiac disease when you have certain specific symptoms and signs with recurrences.

What Happens When You Eat Gluten Containing Food?

When you take a meal containing gluten it will be digested in your stomach and small intestines.

Then the gluten products will enter the cells in your small intestine which is the long tube-like organ that is responsible for digesting and absorbing certain food in your body.

But, in some people, your immune system is making antibodies against these gluten products.

As a result of the action of these antibodies, you will get the symptoms. Mostly these antibodies act on the wall of small intestines leading to the thinning out of the small finger-like projections on the wall called "villi". These villi are important to increase the surface area of absorption of food.

Ultimately when these villi get damaged you will have less surface area to absorb nutrients from food. In turn, this will lead to a lot of complications.

Symptoms and Signs of Gluten Sensitivity

Certainly, you will have nutrient deficiencies due to the poor absorption of them. Such nutrient deficiencies of iron, vitamin B-12, and calcium will cause you to have deficiencies like **anemia**, **vitamin B-12 Deficiency,** and diseases like Osteoporosis.

Other than these, if your children have this condition, they will **not grow adequately for their age**. Similarly, adults will have **weight loss** despite they have meals.

This is due to the lack of absorption of important nutrients as well.

Another important symptom is **long-standing diarrhea**. When your body does not absorb the contents you eat, you will have diarrhea.

On the other hand, specifically, if it doesn't absorb the fat from the diet you consume, then you will have a condition called "Steatorrhea" where you get **bulky and foul-smelling stools**.

Also,

Above all, people will experience **bloating**, **tummy pain**, and sometimes even **heartburn** after consuming a diet containing gluten products.

Besides, recent research found that there is an association of peptic ulcer disease such as heartburn, acid reflux, and stomach ulcers, etc. with gluten sensitivity.

Hence, if you are having long-standing heartburn or acid reflux that would not resolve with the simple medications as it would in other cases, you may have gluten sensitivity!

Other than these, people will have **mouth ulcers**, **inflammation of the tongue**, and **skin conditions** where you get blistering lesions as well.

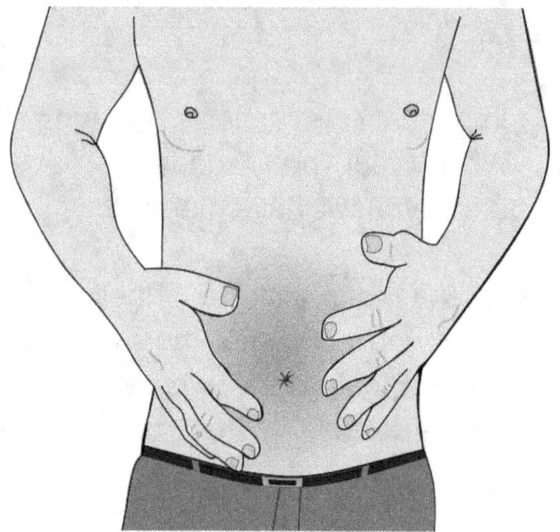

Tummy pain following diet could be due to gluten sensitivity

When to Seek Emergency Medical Help!

Another important point to emphasize is that if the symptoms are very severe, for instance, you can have severe diarrhea and what you eat does not get absorbed; you will have a severe deficiency of nutrients.

Therefore, your body will be very weak and you will have to seek immediate medical attention in this kind of situation. Your doctor will do some tests and will treat you with saline and other medications etc. This condition is called **the "celiac crisis"**.

Consuming a Gluten-Free Diet as a Therapy to Gluten Sensitivity

Consuming a gluten-free diet is the only way you can fight gluten sensitivity. The following steps will aid you to do this.

Know the Contents You Need to Avoid in Your Diet

Mainly, a gluten-free diet includes **NOT** consuming a diet with barley, rye, wheat, and oats.

However, there are some people with gluten sensitivity who report that they consume oats but still, they don't get the symptoms.

This is because although oats are free from gluten naturally, during processing and distribution some other gluten-containing grains get mixed with oats and contaminate them. Anyway, it is better to avoid oats as well if you have the slightest suspicion.

Other than these, while processing and cooking some food, they add gluten-containing products into them. Some of these include hot dogs, candy, modified food starch, French fries, gravy, some salad dressings, sausages, some sauces, thickeners, and vegetables in sauce, etc.

So, though you never eat gluten food still you may have a chance of gluten gets into your body if you consume the above food.

Know What to Eat

Vegetables and fruits, fish, and plain meat do not have any amounts of gluten. However, still, if the aforementioned processing agents are mixed with those, there is a chance of you getting symptoms.

Other than these, grains and flours are safe to consume. Like the same vein, rice, soy, potatoes, beans, millet, corn, eggs, peanuts, butter, and milk are also gluten-free.

Additionally, when it comes to alcoholic beverages, wines, vodka, gin, and gluten-free beers would do the job.

Read the Labels of the Food Items When You are Buying from Supermarkets

It is very important to do this to avoid symptoms. These labels should say the particular food is free from gluten.

And also, if the food contains food processors and additives, it should tell that they are gluten-free. It is safe to avoid such food if those labels do not say that they are gluten-free.

However, if the label says "contains wheat" or similarly, if it contains a specific ingredient like barley, rye, etc. you should avoid that food too.

Conversely, a lot of bread, pasta, etc. preparations available nowadays are gluten-free.

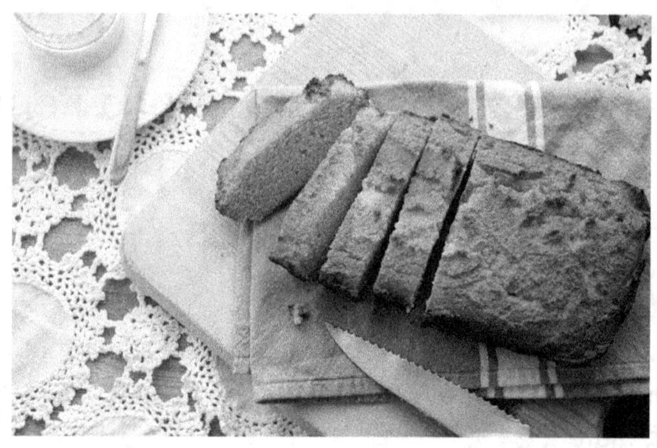

Nowadays lots of products like bread pasta etc.
available as gluten-free preparations

Be Cautious When You Eat at Parties, School, and Other Restaurants, etc.

Although you may not change the circumstances, it is better to ask for a gluten-free menu if available.

On the other hand, you can talk to the chef or the waiter, etc., and ask about the ingredients they used to prepare that meal. If those contain gluten, well, it is better to avoid that food rather than getting into trouble!

Remember that Not Only Food that Contains Gluten

It is not only food that contains gluten but also some medications. When you buy certain medications, the ingredients they put to make the tablet form of the drug may contain gluten.

Most of the time they disclose this information and will tell in the gluten-free label.

However, sometimes they may say that it contains "starch". Since they don't disclose the source of starch, it may come from wheat or corn or whatever.

Needless to say, wheat-containing products are not good for you! So, avoid anything containing starch.

In Conclusion,

To sum up, consuming a gluten-free diet is the only way you can fight gluten sensitivity.

In other words, as far as you don't eat gluten you will be symptom-free. Once you avoid gluten from your diet your intestines will grow back to normal and you will not have any complications.

However, if you have already developed any complications like vitamin B-12 deficiency, anemia, etc. talk to your doctor and your dietitian so that they will help you in managing this condition.

Chapter 8.

Powerful Benefits of Relishing Nutritious King Coconut Water in a Nutshell!

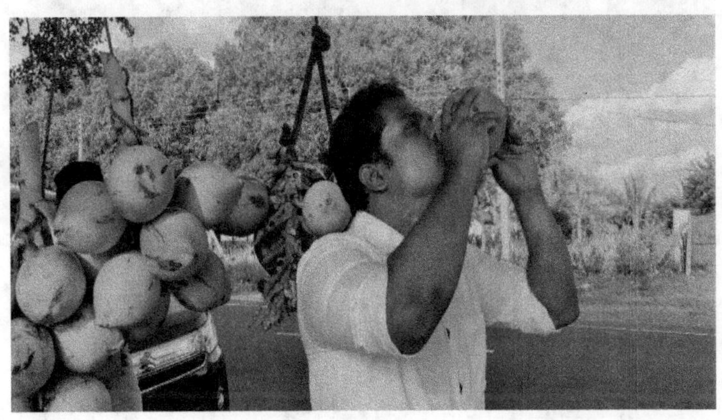

What is King Coconut?

If you are visiting the tropics, relishing nutritious king coconut water is one of the most alluring experiences you should not miss. Other than that, another important thing about king coconut water is that it has tons of health benefits too.

King coconut is a tree mostly similar to coconut which is one of the famous trees in tropical countries. But, due to its golden orange color and the unique taste of its water, it is not wrong to say it's the 'king' of coconuts.

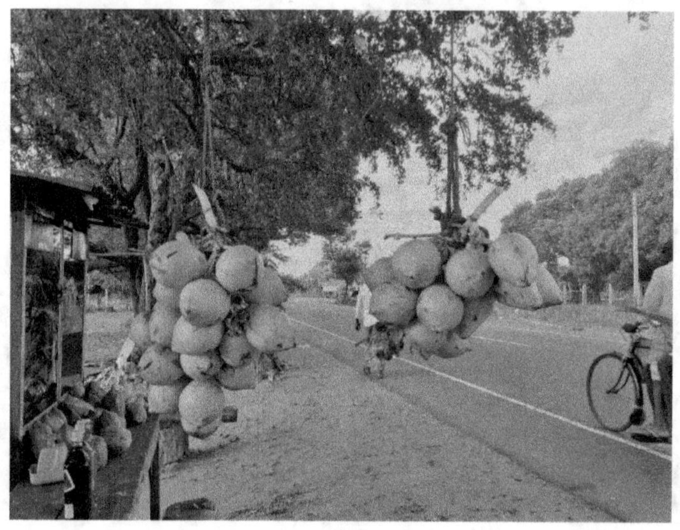

King coconuts selling shops beside the roads in Sri Lanka

Where to Find King Coconuts?

It is an endemic plant for Sri Lanka which a beautiful country in the Indian ocean. Here, almost in any home garden, it's freely available mainly in the village setup. Nevertheless, still, you can see lots of people sell them beside the roads in the urban setting as well. However, some parts of Indonesia have a variety of king coconut, but the taste and color may vary from the original Sri Lankan king coconut.

King coconuts are botanically known as Cocos nucifera var. aurantiaca. Similarly, in the local Sinhalese, they are called 'Thambili'. The palm fruits have been used in local "Ayurvedic" medicine for thousands of years.

Most importantly, unlike the young green coconut, king coconuts are only used for the liquid within. And mainly they have no husk.

Sometimes, local people refer to them as 'coconuts for drinking'. People in Sri Lanka harvest them with extreme care lowering them from the tall palm trees using ropes and pulleys to avoid damaging the precious fruits.

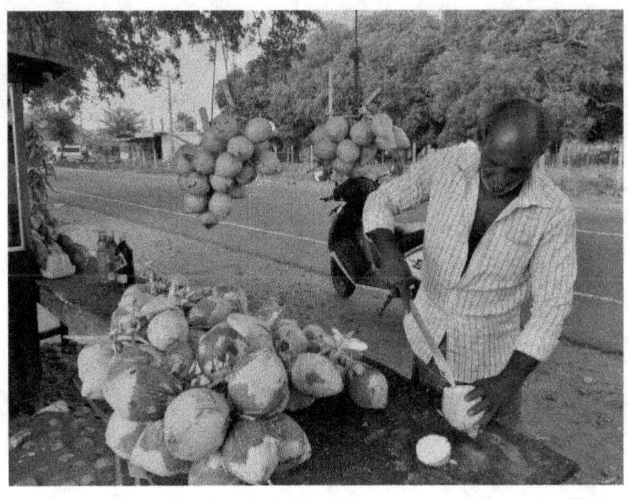

Cutting and preparing fresh king coconut

Health Benefits of Relishing Nutritious King Coconut Water!

Rich in All Nutrients

King coconuts are a rich source of B-complex vitamins including vitamin B-12 and amino acids. Other than that, they have abundant electrolytes which are minerals like potassium, calcium, sodium, magnesium, chloride, and phosphate.

Above all, the liquid within the King coconuts not only has more magnesium and calcium than an orange but also more potassium than a banana.

Likewise, the king coconuts are a rich source of carbohydrates, vitamin E, iron, calcium, and phosphorous. Besides, it also has a high dietary soluble fiber and appreciable amounts of protein and fat.

Certainly, considering all of this needless to say the king coconut is a wonder that has a cure for almost every ailment.

Excellent Natural Solution to Prevent Dehydration

It will naturally replenish the body's loss of electrolytes by sweating during exercise or any other type of exertion. Subsequently, this helps prevent dehydration and fatigue.

Compared to the aerated waters that are usually artificially colored and flavored, the natural coconut drink refreshes and purifies the body. So, in your daily exercise session, use king coconut water to stay hydrated.

It contains a high amount of potassium and sodium. In other words, electrolyte levels close to that of human plasma. Therefore, it makes an excellent re-hydrant. Moreover, this makes it a great way to prevent muscle cramps while remaining a great and natural energy boost.

Aids in Digestion, Gastrointestinal, and Urinary Tract Disease

King coconuts contain bio-active enzymes that aid in digestion and help with the body's metabolism. The liquid contains trace amounts of natural sucrose, fructose, and glucose.

That is to say, it is effective in treating gastrointestinal diseases, useful in treating cholera, improves constipation as well as being effective in treating diarrhea in babies too.

Drinking a glass of king Coconut water every morning both prevents and remedies intestinal worms in children. Moms! Include it in your morning smoothie and incorporate it into your child's breakfast.

Children are more prone to urinary tract infections than adults. King Coconut water acts as a diuretic meanwhile the nutritious water effectively flushes out infections from the bladder and urinary tract.

However, heating or any type of temperature pasteurization can reduce the nutritional benefits of King coconut water.

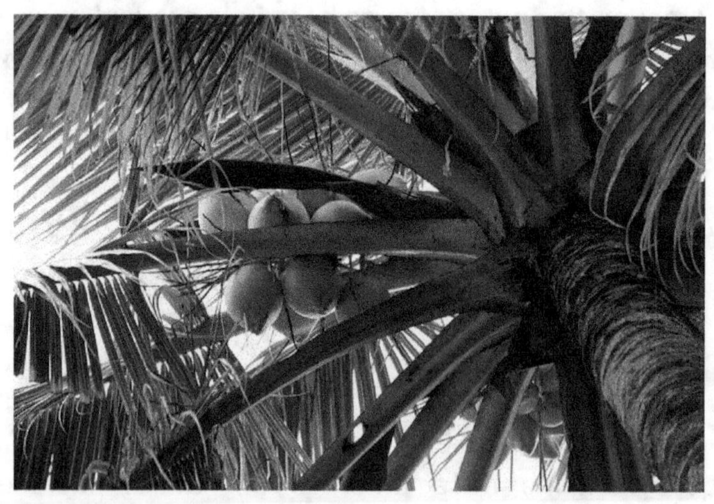

Improves Skin Health

King coconut oil is a local product that is famous among traditional "Ayurvedic" medics when applied locally promotes hair growth.

Drinking king coconut water moisturizes skin from within and eliminates any excess oil.

Similarly, it contains anti-bacterial and anti-viral properties that help cure skin infections effectively thus helping your skin remain clean, clear, and healthy.

It is a Powerful Antioxidant and an Antidote

Moreover, king coconut water is also an effective antidote to counteract the strong side effects that some modern drugs may have on the body. Besides, studies have found the water has antioxidant properties too.

In many Sri Lankan "Ayurvedic" remedies, the king coconut has a great place to cure many ailments related to impurities in the system.

Beware!

However, some studies reported that people with certain diseases should alarm themselves while consuming excessive amounts of king coconut water.

For instance, if you are suffering from diabetes, chronic renal impairment, and potassium retaining medication, there is a high risk of developing "hyperkalemia" which is a condition where you get excessive potassium levels in the blood if you consume too much. This is due to its high potassium content.

But don't worry.

If you are suffering from any of these diseases consult your doctor and take advice. With your doctor's advice, still you can consume and enjoy the benefits of this amazing natural product.

In Conclusion,

To sum up, king coconut water has tons of health benefits.

Relishing nutritious king coconut water is a must. There are a lot of commercial preparations of king coconut water now available in the market.

But, needless to say, not only its benefits but also the pure enjoyment it gives when you consume it naturally from the fruit. Don't forget to enjoy this fruit on your next trip to the tropics!

About the Author

Dr. Pasindu Abeysundara is a medical practitioner from Sri Lanka. He is interested in sharing his knowledge in medicine with the general public in a simplified and easy-to-understand manner. Further, he believes in the prevention of disease is better than cure.

He was graduated from the University of Peradeniya in Sri Lanka with an MBBS degree and has the experience of treating patients in the fields of Medicine, Surgery, and Psychiatry for years in various parts of Sri Lanka.

To visit his website, type the following in your web browser.

https://healthfactsbydoctorpasindu.com/

Next,

Other Books by the Author

3 Strategies of Managing Stress

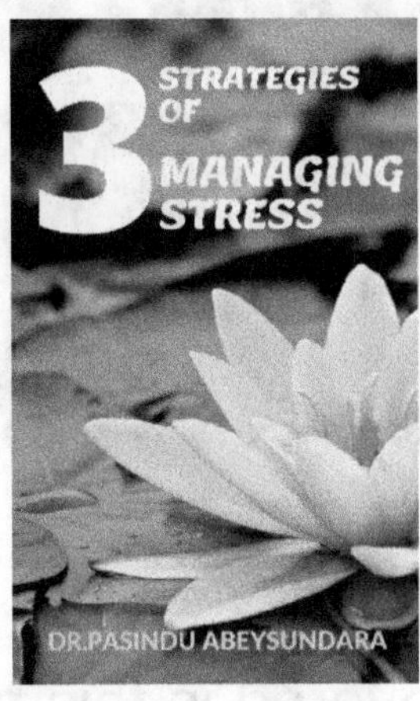

Topics covered in this book are,

Strategy No. 1 – Understanding the Cause and Effect

Strategy No. 2 – Practicing Mindfulness

Strategy No. 3 – Practicing a Relaxation Exercise

Healthy Lifestyle Hacks

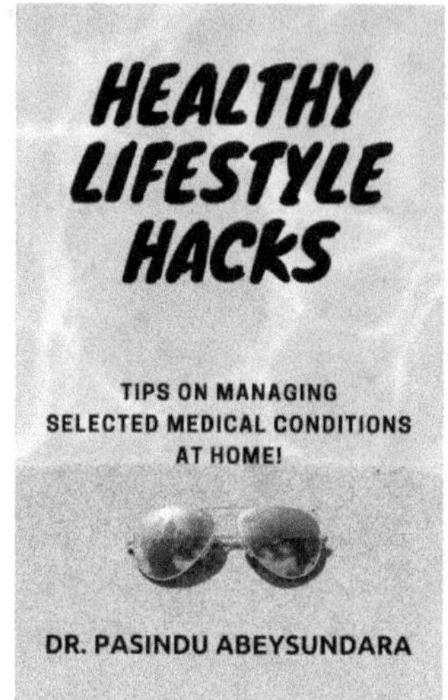

<u>Topics covered in this book are,</u>

1. How to Treat a LIGAMENT SPRAIN at Home!
2. How to Treat the UPPER BACK PAIN due to RHOMBOID SPASMS at Home!
3. How to Treat DRY EYES at Home!
4. How to Treat the HEEL PAIN due to PLANTAR FASCIITIS, at Home!
5. How to TAKE CARE of a BEDBOUND PERSON at Home!

Healthy Lifestyle Hacks 02

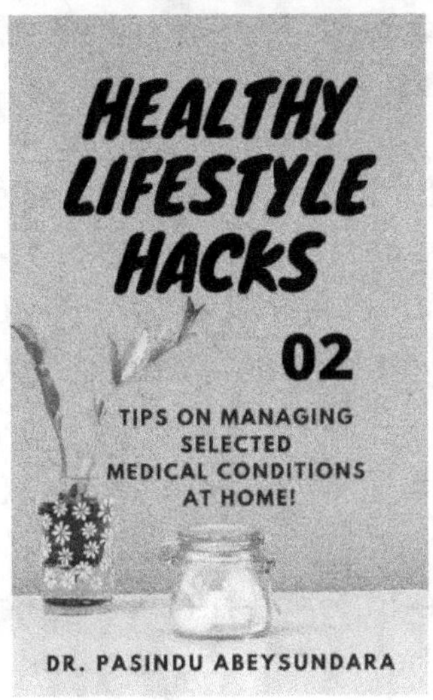

Topics covered in this book are;

Chapter 01 - Managing the Pain of Osteoarthritis at Home

Chapter 02 - Understanding Osteoporosis and Preventive Measures

Chapter 03 - Diabetic Foot Care

Chapter 04 - Maintaining better Postures is very Important!

Chapter 05 - Managing some Specific Causes of Headache

One Last Thing!

If you enjoyed this book or found it to be useful, I would be grateful if you could post a short review on Amazon. Your support does make a big difference. And I read all the reviews personally so I can get your feedback and make this writing experience even better.

If you would like to leave a review, then all you need to do is click the review button link on this book's page on Amazon.

Thanks again for your support!

Dr. Pasindu Abeysundara.